THE BOOK OF

MINDFULNESS

LIZZIE CORNWALL

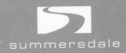

summersdale

THE BOOK OF MINDFULNESS

Copyright © Summersdale Publishers Ltd, 2015

Research by Katherine Bassford

All rights reserved.

No part of this book may be reproduced by any means, nor transmitted, nor translated into a machine language, without the written permission of the publishers.

Condition of Sale
This book is sold subject to the condition that it shall not, by way of trade or otherwise, be lent, re-sold, hired out or otherwise circulated in any form of binding or cover other than that in which it is published and without a similar condition including this condition being imposed on the subsequent purchaser.

Summersdale Publishers Ltd
46 West Street
Chichester
West Sussex
PO19 1RP
UK

www.summersdale.com

Printed and bound in China

ISBN: 978-1-84953-655-4

Substantial discounts on bulk quantities of Summersdale books are available to corporations, professional associations and other organisations. For details contact Nicky Douglas by telephone: +44 (0) 1243 756902, fax: +44 (0) 1243 786300 or email: nicky@summersdale.com.

To...

From...

Be happy in the moment, that's enough. Each moment is all we need, not more.

Mother Teresa

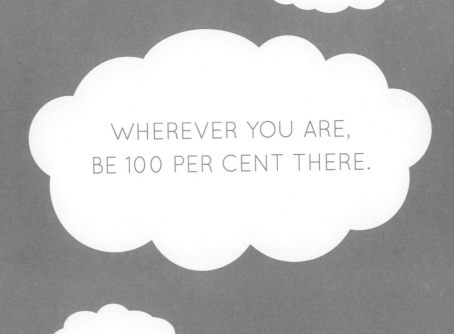

WHEREVER YOU ARE,
BE 100 PER CENT THERE.

HAPPINESS IS A
JOURNEY, NOT A
DESTINATION.

Do every act of your life as
if it were your last.

Marcus Aurelius

The greatest step towards a life of simplicity is to learn to let go.

Steve Maraboli

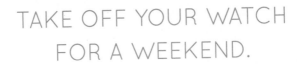

TAKE OFF YOUR WATCH
FOR A WEEKEND.

CALM BREATH. CALM
MIND. CALM MOMENT.

To see a world in a grain of sand,
And heaven in a wild flower,
Hold infinity in the palm of your hand,
And eternity in an hour.

William Blake

When you realise there is nothing lacking, the whole world belongs to you.

Lao Tzu

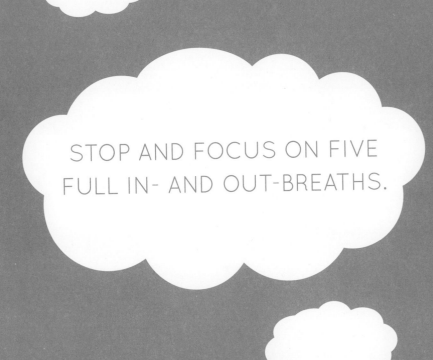

STOP AND FOCUS ON FIVE FULL IN- AND OUT-BREATHS.

PLACE LITTLE NOTES
AROUND YOUR HOME OR
WORKSPACE TO REMIND YOU
TO 'PAUSE' AND 'BREATHE'.

You're only here for a short visit. Don't hurry, don't worry. And be sure to smell the flowers along the way.

Walter Hagen

We have more possibilities
available in each moment
than we realise.

Thích Nhất Hạnh

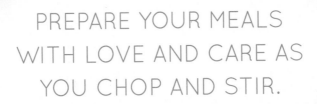

PREPARE YOUR MEALS WITH LOVE AND CARE AS YOU CHOP AND STIR.

THE PURPOSE OF LIFE
IS TO ENJOY IT.

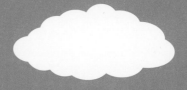

The greatest weapon
against stress is our ability
to choose one thought
over another.

William James

Paradise is not a place; it is a state of consciousness.

Sri Chinmoy

GIVE YOURSELF
EXTRA TIME TO GET TO
PLACES – SO YOU CAN SLOW
DOWN AND ARRIVE
MINDFULLY.

INSTRUCTION FOR LIFE:
PAY ATTENTION.

Every breath we take,
every step we make, can
be filled with peace, joy
and serenity.

Thích Nhất Hạnh

We have only now,
only this single eternal moment
opening and unfolding before
us, day and night.

Jack Kornfield

OBSERVE YOUR THOUGHTS
AS THEY COME AND GO; LET
THEM PASS BY LIKE CLOUDS
IN THE SKY.

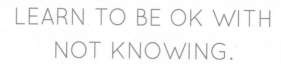

LEARN TO BE OK WITH
NOT KNOWING.

In the midst of movement
and chaos, keep stillness
inside of you.

Deepak Chopra

Mindfulness means being awake. It means knowing what you are doing.

Jon Kabat-Zinn

WHEN YOU WASH
YOUR HANDS, PAY ATTENTION
TO THE WATER ON YOUR
SKIN AND THE SCENT
OF THE SOAP.

THE MOMENT YOU
ACCEPT YOURSELF
JUST AS YOU ARE IS
THE MOMENT YOU
FIND PEACE.

For fast-acting relief,
try slowing down.

Lily Tomlin

You don't have to be
swept away by your feeling...
respond with wisdom and kindness
rather than habit and reactivity.

Bhante Henepola Gunaratana

LOOK AT EVERYTHING
AS THOUGH YOU WERE
SEEING IT FOR THE
FIRST TIME.

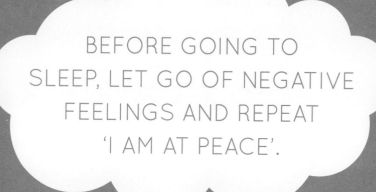

BEFORE GOING TO
SLEEP, LET GO OF NEGATIVE
FEELINGS AND REPEAT
'I AM AT PEACE'.

Peace comes from within.
Do not seek it without.

Buddha

We can always
begin again.

Jack Kornfield

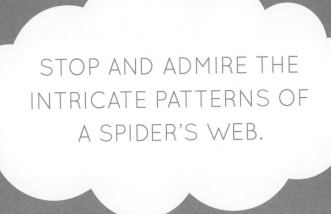

STOP AND ADMIRE THE
INTRICATE PATTERNS OF
A SPIDER'S WEB.

WHEN OUR MINDS ARE
ENGULFED IN WORRIES,
WE ARE MISSING THE
EXPERIENCE OF
THE MOMENT.

Drink your tea slowly and reverently, as if it is the axis on which the world earth revolves.

Thích Nhất Hạnh

Time is not a line, but a
series of now-points.

Taisen Deshimaru

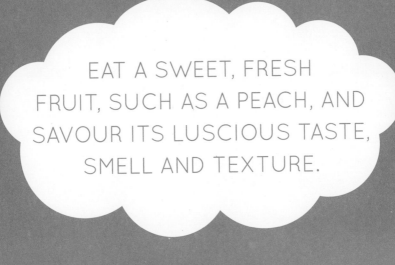

EAT A SWEET, FRESH FRUIT, SUCH AS A PEACH, AND SAVOUR ITS LUSCIOUS TASTE, SMELL AND TEXTURE.

START TO NOTICE
WHICH EXPERIENCES AND
PEOPLE ENERGISE YOU, AND
WHICH DRAIN YOU.

Only loving-kindness and right-mindfulness can free us.

Maha Ghosananda

The wise man is
a happy child.

Arnaud Desjardins

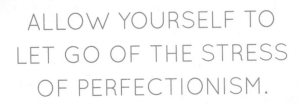

ALLOW YOURSELF TO
LET GO OF THE STRESS
OF PERFECTIONISM.

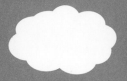

LEARNING SOMETHING
NEW HELPS BRING
YOU FULLY INTO
THE PRESENT.

The most difficult times for many of us are the ones we give ourselves.

Pema Chödrön

If you wait for tomorrow, tomorrow comes. If you don't wait for tomorrow, tomorrow comes.

Senegalese proverb

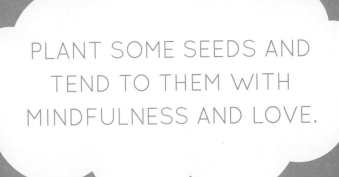

PLANT SOME SEEDS AND
TEND TO THEM WITH
MINDFULNESS AND LOVE.

BE A COMPASSIONATE
FRIEND TO YOURSELF.

Forever – is
composed of Nows.

Emily Dickinson

Have a mind that is
open to everything, and
attached to nothing.

Tilopa

AFTER ANY ACHIEVEMENT, PRAISE YOURSELF BEFORE RUSHING ON TO THE NEXT CHALLENGE.

LOOK FOR THE BEST
IN EVERYONE!

The mind... can be compared to the sky, covered by layers of cloud which hide its true nature.

Kalu Rinpoche

The trees that are slow to grow bear the best fruit.

Molière

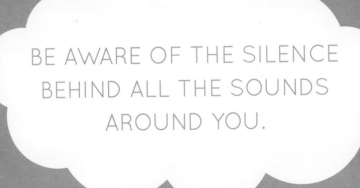

BE AWARE OF THE SILENCE
BEHIND ALL THE SOUNDS
AROUND YOU.

BY BEING HAPPY IN
THIS MOMENT YOU
ARE CREATING MORE
HAPPINESS.

If you want to conquer
the anxiety of life, live in the
moment, live in the breath.

Amit Ray

Whatever the present
moment contains, accept it
as if you had chosen it.

Eckhart Tolle

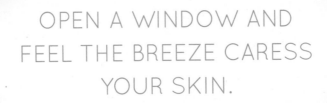

OPEN A WINDOW AND
FEEL THE BREEZE CARESS
YOUR SKIN.

THERE IS JOY IN
JUST BEING.

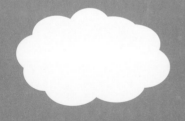

If you want to be
happy, be so.

Kozma Petrovich Prutkov

Knowledge is learning something every day. Wisdom is letting go of something every day.

Zen proverb

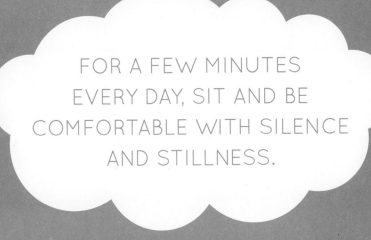

FOR A FEW MINUTES
EVERY DAY, SIT AND BE
COMFORTABLE WITH SILENCE
AND STILLNESS.

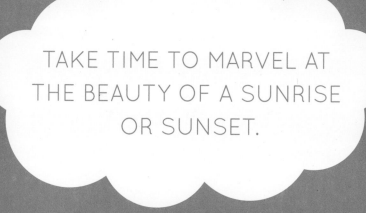

TAKE TIME TO MARVEL AT THE BEAUTY OF A SUNRISE OR SUNSET.

Everything you do can
be done better from a
place of relaxation.

Stephen C. Paul

It is very simple to
be happy, but it is very
difficult to be simple.

Rabindranath Tagore

SPEND TIME WITH CHILDREN. THEY SEE MAGIC AND WONDER IN EVERYDAY THINGS AND LIVE IN THE PRESENT MOMENT.

LIFE HAPPENS.
LET IT BE.

How much of your life do
you spend looking forward to
being somewhere else?

Matthew Flickstein

Life is denied by lack
of attention, whether it be to
cleaning windows or trying to
write a masterpiece.

Nadia Boulanger

WHEN WAITING IN A
QUEUE, FOCUS ON THE CONTACT
YOUR FEET MAKE WITH THE FLOOR
AND ENJOY THE FEELING OF BEING
GROUNDED AND SUPPORTED.

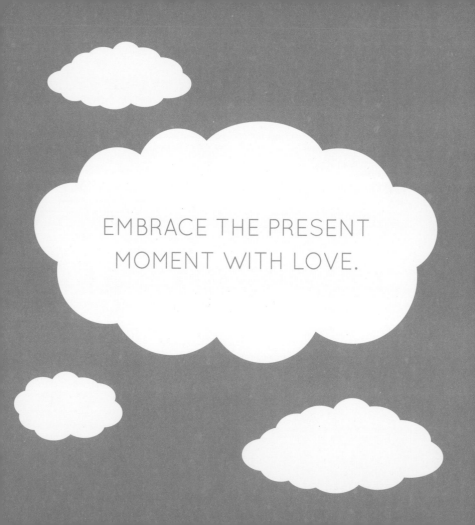

EMBRACE THE PRESENT
MOMENT WITH LOVE.

Mindful time spent with
the person we love is the
fullest expression of true love
and real generosity.

Thích Nhất Hạnh

Those who are always preoccupied with something cannot enjoy the world.

Lao Tzu

MEDITATE WHILE
CLEANING OR WASHING
UP BY FOCUSING ON EVERY
SENSORY DETAIL.

NOTICE THE DIFFERENT SOUNDS AROUND YOU AND PRACTISE BEING OPEN TO ALL SOUNDS, WHEREVER THEY ARISE.

Get out of your head
and get into your heart.
Think less, feel more.

Osho

Learning how to be
still, to really be still and let
life happen – that stillness
becomes a radiance.

Morgan Freeman

GO BAREFOOT ON
THE BEACH OR IN THE PARK
AND ENJOY THE DIFFERENT
TEXTURES BENEATH
YOUR FEET.

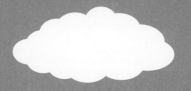

LIFE IS LIVED TODAY, NOT TOMORROW.

To live fully is to let go and
die with each passing moment...
to be reborn in each new one.

Jack Kornfield

Never be afraid to sit
a while and think.

Lorraine Hansberry

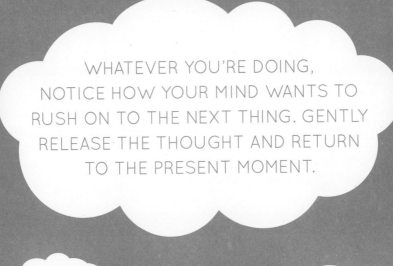

WHATEVER YOU'RE DOING, NOTICE HOW YOUR MIND WANTS TO RUSH ON TO THE NEXT THING. GENTLY RELEASE THE THOUGHT AND RETURN TO THE PRESENT MOMENT.

EVERYTHING HAPPENS
FOR A REASON.

A crust eaten in peace
is better than a banquet
partaken in anxiety.

Aesop

It's good to have an end
in mind, but in the end what
counts is how you travel.

Orna Ross

SIT IN A CAFE OR ON A
PARK BENCH AND SEND LOVE
TO EVERYONE AROUND YOU.
REMEMBER WE ARE ALL
CONNECTED.

WAITING IS AN
OPPORTUNITY FOR
MINDFULNESS.

Mindful eating is a
way to become reacquainted
with the guidance of our
internal nutritionist.

Jan Chozen Bays

Sit. Be still. And listen.

Rumi

VISUALISE YOUR BREATH
FILLING YOUR BODY WITH
HEALING WHITE LIGHT.

URGES WILL COME AND
GO. YOU DON'T HAVE
TO ACT ON THEM.

Nature does not hurry, yet everything is accomplished.

Lao Tzu

It is only possible to
live happily ever after on
a day-to-day basis.

Margaret Wander Bonanno

SEE HOW SLOWLY
AND SOFTLY YOU CAN DO
THINGS TODAY AND ENJOY
THE PEACE THIS BRINGS.

COME HOME TO
THE PRESENT.

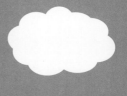

Nowhere can man find
a quieter or more untroubled
retreat than in his own soul.

Marcus Aurelius

We live in the world
when we love it.

Rabindranath Tagore

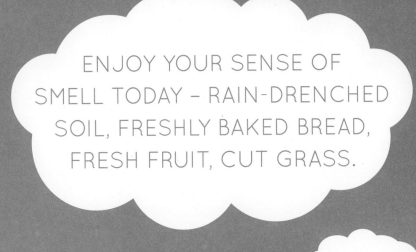

ENJOY YOUR SENSE OF SMELL TODAY – RAIN-DRENCHED SOIL, FRESHLY BAKED BREAD, FRESH FRUIT, CUT GRASS.

ALL WORDS CONTAIN
ENERGY AND VIBRATION.
SPEAK FROM A PLACE
OF LOVE.

Do you have the patience to wait till your mud settles and the water is clear? Can you remain unmoving till the right action arises by itself?

Lao Tzu

We are what we think.
All that we are arises with our
thoughts. With our thoughts
we make our world.

Buddha

WHEN THE PHONE RINGS,
TAKE ONE MINDFUL BREATH
BEFORE ANSWERING.

THE ORDINARY CAN BE
EXTRAORDINARY.

For peace of mind,
we need to resign as general
manager of the universe.

Larry Eisenberg

The point of mindfulness is not to get rid of thought but to learn to see thought skilfully.

Jack Kornfield

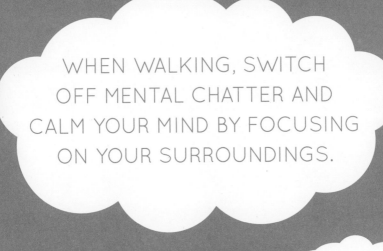

WHEN WALKING, SWITCH OFF MENTAL CHATTER AND CALM YOUR MIND BY FOCUSING ON YOUR SURROUNDINGS.

WE ARRIVE HERE WITH
NOTHING AND WE
LEAVE WITH NOTHING.

Your mind is your instrument.
Learn to be its master
and not its slave.

Remez Sasson

Change your thoughts and you change your world.

Norman Vincent Peale

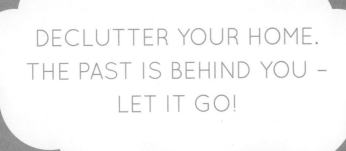

DECLUTTER YOUR HOME.
THE PAST IS BEHIND YOU –
LET IT GO!

LIKE CLOUDS IN THE
SKY, EVERYTHING IS IN
A CONSTANT PROCESS
OF CHANGE.

Don't let yesterday use up
too much of today.

Cherokee proverb

Mindfulness isn't difficult,
we just need to remember
to do it.

Sharon Salzberg

THROUGHOUT THE DAY,
LOOK FOR THINGS TO BE
THANKFUL FOR – A HOT
SHOWER, THE BIRDS OUTSIDE,
FRESH FOOD.

LIFE IS A CYCLE OF
ENDINGS AND NEW
BEGINNINGS.

Once you stop clinging
and let things be, you'll be free, even
of birth and death. You'll transform
everything... And you'll be at
peace wherever you are.

Bodhidharma

Meditation practice isn't about trying to throw ourselves away or become something better. It's about befriending who we are already.

Pema Chödrön

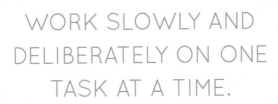

WORK SLOWLY AND
DELIBERATELY ON ONE
TASK AT A TIME.

DO NOT MISS YOUR APPOINTMENT WITH LIFE.

One joy scatters a
hundred griefs.

Chinese proverb

Happiness arises in a state of peace, not of tumult.

Ann Radcliffe

WHEN TRAVELLING BY TRAIN OR BUS, TURN OFF YOUR MOBILE AND LOOK OUT AT THE VIEW.

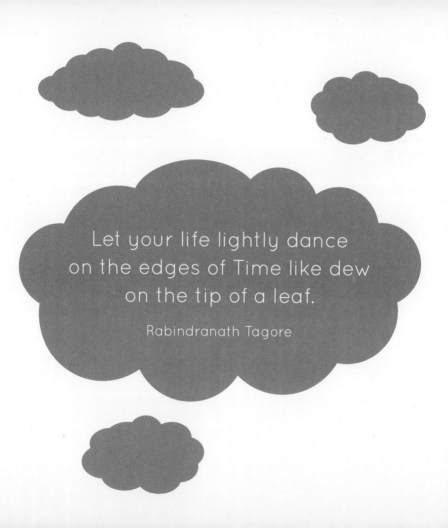

Let your life lightly dance
on the edges of Time like dew
on the tip of a leaf.

Rabindranath Tagore

Walk as if you
are kissing the earth
with your feet.

Thích Nhất Hạnh

If you're interested in finding out more about our books,
find us on Facebook at **Summersdale Publishers** and
follow us on Twitter at **@Summersdale**.

www.summersdale.com